The Newest
Weight Watchers Freestyle Zero Point Cookbook

70 Low Point Recipes, 7-Day Freestyle Weight Loss Meal Plan, Lose Up to 10 Pounds in 1 Week

By Dr. Emma Green

Table of Contents

Book Description

Without any doubt, Weight Watchers Freestyle cookbook is a smart approach to lose weight. With more than 200 food items with zero Smart Points, this diet will be a complete game changer. The new list has lots of surprises for you. This plan allows you to lose weight without starving.

We have drafted this book for your assistance. In this book, you will find essentials of this new program, list of food items with zero SmartPoints and 70 delicious recipes. With a 7-day freestyle weight loss meal plan, it will be easy for you to plan your diet within your allocated SmartPoints. This book covers:

- Essential of Weight Watchers Freestyle Program
- Sample Meal Plan
- Ideas to Increase Your Success Chances
- Delicious Recipes for Breakfast, Dinner, and Lunch
- Healthy Snacks and Dessert Recipes
- 10 bonus recipes for your journey

Get ready to start a healthy life without any trouble and compromise. A new opportunity with lots of perks is waiting for you.

Introduction

Are you tired of weight loss programs and strict diet? Do you want to eat plenty of food even while shedding your extra pounds? Congratulation, Weight Watchers has made a significant switch from PointsPlus to revolutionary SmartPoints. The new Weight Watchers Freestyle plan is designed in a way to control your overeating.

The new program works completely different than the concept of calories. When you consider the impact of food on the body, calories will tell only a half story. A cookie contains 100 calories, but the cookies lack nutrients. On the other hand, 100 calories of vegetables, tofu, and turkey offer more nutrients. Counting calories without considering nutrients will not help you to follow a healthy diet. Nutrients are essential to decrease the risk of diseases and promote healthy weight loss.

If you are interested to know more about this plan, this book must be the perfect choice for you. To make this book a complete guide for you, we have included healthy WW Freestyle recipes, which will help you to reduce weight and maintain a healthy body.

The book has a complete list of zero point food so that you can easily include healthy food items in your diet to stay healthy and full.

Chapter 1 – Essentials of Weight Watchers Freestyle Program

The Weight Watchers Freestyle programs are based on extremely effective SmartPoints System. It is even more beneficial than previous programs.

Essential Rules and Cautions of Weight Watchers Freestyle

Freestyle is a bold step of allocating zero points to more than 200 foods like tofu, lentils, peas, beans, plain yogurt without fat, turkey breast without skin, chicken breast without skin, seafood, fish, corn, and eggs. These foods don't a necessity to be measured or tracker. This smart change is based on lifestyle and nutritional research. It allows unprecedented levels of freedom to lose weight.

SmartPoints focus on previous the consumption of healthy food instead of weight loss. SmartPoints combine complex nutritional details. This particular number proves helpful for members to move toward fruit, vegetables, and lean proteins while avoiding saturated fat and sugar.

In the previous program, all carbs had same treatment in a formula. The emphasis on sugar is significant. Fortunately, most vegetables and all fresh fruits are zero SmartPoints.

Individualized Plan

Weekly and daily points of members will be adjusted as per the metabolic rate of the individual. The programs start with a personalized assessment capturing the goals and lifestyle information. It is a customized program of Weight Watcher to date.

Activity and Fitness

Beyond the weighing scale, there is a new attitude and approach toward exercises. Each member obtains personalized activity goals. Whether you want to get active or not, this is a core part of this new program.

Meetings and Connect of Weight Watchers

In-person conferences have had upgrades with more focus on goals both off and the scale. It is a part of a holistic approach than focusing on diet and weight. Connect is a community platform that conveys the community closer for joint support.

App Overhaul

The weight watcher app is around, but it is now improved for Freestyle weight watchers program. FitBreak is a new app to integrate with the current app. It inspires users to take fitbreaks throughout their day and currently have more than 70 inspirational options.

This a practical and welcome upgrade to Weight Watchers program. People are considering healthy, and natural food and Weight Watchers has adjusted this points system for their assistance.

The focus of this program is goals of your lifestyle, and it is a wise move. There is nothing called a "diet" in segregation. Your lifestyle choices always influence your way to eat and play an essential role in sustainable programs for weight management.

Follow Your SmartPoints Budget

Your regular SmartPoints indicate the number of points that you will spend on drinks and food regularly. It is personalized for each person based on the gender, age, weight, and height. If you want to get desired results, you must get the exact amount of healthy nutrients.

You will get the weekly points to spend regularly and save them for special occasions. There is no need to consume all points and use them carefully. The points reset at the start of each week.

You should choose foods with lower SmartPoints like veggies, fruits, whole grains and lean proteins. It will increase your SmartPoints and direct you toward healthy choices.

How does Weight Watchers Freestyle Work?

Each drink and food has SmartPoints value. It is an easy-to-use number based on protein, sugar, saturated fat and calories. You will get a SmartPoints budget that pushes you to make a healthy eating choice while noticing weight loss results and staying satisfied.

Their zero points category of food contains vegetables, fruits, and lean proteins. These food items offer a foundation from which a person can build healthy eating pattern without imposing a risk of overeating. It is easy to see when you are feeling satisfied instead of overeating them. It can be hard to each six chicken breasts instead of six cookies.

Freestyle Smart Points Calculation

The purpose of this program is to help you reach your desired weight without starving. Weight watchers freestyle helps you to develop a healthy relationship with food. The whole program is based on the calculation of SmartPoints. This SmartPoints system is science-based and assigns a number to each food as per four components, protein, sugar, saturated fat and calories. The higher figure shows that the food has more saturated fat and sugar. The lower value of food indicates that the food has less saturated fat and sugar and more protein.

The calculation of SmartPoints is the latest method of Weight Watchers to make a smart selection. The FreeStyle Plan of Weight Watchers is introduced in January 2018. However, there are some changes; this new program still uses SmartPoints. With SmartPoints program, before and after the introduction of Freestyle, the regular allowance is independently determined. There is no particular formula because each person has different priorities. You have to remember your weekly and daily allowance.

Previously, the least daily allowance was 26 points. The lowest daily allowance for Freestyle program is 23. The current contribution is low because they have introduced different foods with zero points. The weekly allowance may vary for every person so make sure to get this at first meeting or online tools of WW.

Weight Watchers has modified the way to give points to food with different calculations and plan with PointsPlus system, the nutritive values were total fat, protein, fiber, and carbs. Before this, WW utilized calories fiber and fat to determine the amounts of food.

Plan of Weight Watcher allows you to make lifelong changes in your eating habits. The new calculation will enable you to choose right food and stay healthy. The latest calculation method includes the use of following nutritional values:

❖ Protein
❖ Sugar
❖ Saturated Fat
❖ Calories

The weight or value given to each factor varies. For example, saturated fat has a higher value than calories. Sugar will cause a high point value because it provides a significant factor than calories.

Protein can decrease the value of points while calculation of SmartPoints so higher protein food means lower points value it has. A meal may have similar value for protein and calories, but if saturated fat or sugar is higher in these items. Give different values to each piece in the calculation may guide you to choose healthy food items though both have a similar number of calories.

Smart Points Food Value Calculation

(Calories * .0305) + (Saturated Fat * .275) + (Sugar * .12) – (Protein * .098)

Before SmartPoints, the plan was a point plush calculation. See the Points Plus calculations to understand the difference.

(Fat (g) / 3.8889) + (Carbohydrate (g) / 9.2105) + (Protein (g) / 10.9375) – (Fiber (g) /12.5)

The higher content of sugar in food can double the value. In this formula, the carbs were in plus method (that is high because of sugars) it is difficult to determine if these were bad or good carbs.

By utilizing sugar instead of carbs, the values will guide you to healthy foods and carbs. While numerous food items have a high value with SmartPoints calculation. The new plan allows you to get higher weekly and daily allowance than the old method.

It is difficult to calculate certain allowance because it is an individual evaluation. You can be a member of Weight Watchers Freestyle to get your personal allowance.

The Difference Between the New and Old WW Program

May things are same, such as SmartPoints are still an essential part of this plan. You can earn points for activities and plan steers you toward healthy choices. Weight Watchers (WW) Freestyle is launched with some changes. Before you start following WW freestyle, you must know all essential details, such as a new list of zero point foods.

Vegetables

Most fruits and vegetables are zero points on WW, even on previous plans. They are still there with some additions. Peas and sweet corn are a part of this list. It is exciting news for the lovers of sweet corn and peas.

Another exciting change in the veggie world of WW is the presence of starchy veggies on this list. It includes lentils and beans. Food items like pinto beans, black beans, and chickpeas are foods with zero points.

If you want to buy a canned version, make sure to choose a can without added sugar and oil. You have to calculate the Freestyle Smart Points based on the nutrition details on the label. You can use WW mobile application to verify the nutrients in canned food.

What is not in zero point list?

While there are some vegetables to this zero points list of WW Freestyle program, but some vegetables are not on the list. These include dried veggies and snacks that are easy to overeat. Potatoes are not on the list because this starchy vegetable is natural to over-consume.

Meats

The old programs of Weight Watchers don't have meats in the list of zero point foods. It is the biggest change for people because the list has some lean meats like turkey and chicken. The freestyle plan allows you to have lean turkey and chicken breast. It should be skinless to add it to the list of zero points food.

Lean turkey breast and chicken breast meats have zero value. You may have ground lean chicken and turkey without any trouble. If you are using these items in your recipe, the recipe calculator of Weight Watchers can calculate the value of these foods. If you can calculate these points, make sure to remove the nourishment value for turkey and chicken.

Meats that are not in Zero List

You can't include lean beef and pork in your diet because these are not on this list. As per healthy diet recommendations, you have to limit the consumption of red meat in each week. The WW freestyle requires you to encourage healthy foods. The red meats have a particular point value. Moreover, dried meat like jerky is not zero. You can easily overeat these snacks. These are not in the list of WW freestyle.

Seafood and Fish

All seafood and fish are available in the zero Freestyle Smart Points list of WW freestyle program. Some seafood and fish are high in fats, but you can get them on the list. The reason is their beneficial nutrients. The healthy diet always encourages the consumption of seafood and fish for their nutrients.

You should buy fresh seafood and avoid canned items with added oil. You can choose a fish in water instead of oil. With WW mobile app, you can quickly scan the label of the food to verify points.

What is not available in the category?

Even though all seafood and fish are on this list, but canned versions are prohibited. Just like dried meat, the dried fish items don't have zero points. Smoked fish may be useful like smoked turkey and chicken breasts.

Fruits

There is nothing special to mention in this category. The fruits with zero points in old plans are still in the new list. You must avoid canned fruits with added sugars and oil. Plantains and Avocados are not on the zero points list of WW freestyle.

Moreover, if you are making smoothies with the food items on the zero point list, still you have to calculate its Freestyle Smart Points. The reason is that the vegetables or fruits are in liquid form and you can eat more yogurt and fruits without feeling full. Therefore, it is necessary to track your points.

New Foods

Other food items on the Freestyle list are eggs, plain yogurt without fat, Quorn, meat substitute, and tofu. There are several reasons to add these food items on the list, such as promote healthy eating and nutritional benefits. While grabbing a yogurt from the shelf, make sure to consider its fat content. You should choose unsweetened plain and nonfat yogurt. If you are consuming sweetened yogurt, you must track and calculate the points.

The list doesn't have cottage cheese or soft cheese. These may be high in calories, and people can consume more of these food items than yogurt.

Other Changes in WW Freestyle

While the latest zero points food items are the main changes, there are other important things for your weight loss goal. Your regular unused points will roll over in the subsequent day (almost 4 points). The procedure continues during the week and allows the rollover to go from a day to another.

If you don't use these rolled over points at the conclusion of the week, these will go away. These will not roll in the next week. You can bank these points in extras along with some weekly points. You can use these points for a particular day.

Full List of Zero Point Foods

With a list of zero point foods to choose from, you will get something delicious to eat. Here is a complete list of zero point foods.

- ❖ Apples
- ❖ Unsweetened applesauce
- ❖ Arrowroot
- ❖ Apricots
- ❖ Artichoke hearts and Artichokes
- ❖ Asparagus
- ❖ Arugula
- ❖ Banana
- ❖ Bamboo shoots

- ❖ Beans, including white, wax, string, soy, snap, small white, pink, navy, mung, lupine, lima, kidney, great norther, chickpeas (garbanzo), green, Roman Cranberry, cannellini, butter, fava broad, black and adzuki
- ❖ Fat-free, refined and canned Beans
- ❖ Mixed Berries
- ❖ Beets
- ❖ Blueberries
- ❖ Blackberries
- ❖ Broccoli rabe
- ❖ Broccoli
- ❖ Broccolini
- ❖ Broccoli Slaw
- ❖ Brussels sprouts
- ❖ Cabbage of all varieties like pickled, savory, napa, red, green, Japanese and bok choy
- ❖ Grilled Calamari
- ❖ Carrots
- ❖ Cantaloupe
- ❖ Cauliflower
- ❖ Celery
- ❖ Caviar
- ❖ Swiss chard
- ❖ Ground Chicken breast (fat-free)
- ❖ Cherries
- ❖ Tenderloin or Chicken boneless, skinless and with bones
- ❖ Collards
- ❖ Clementines coleslaw blend (carrots and shredded cabbage), packed
- ❖ Corn and baby corns, yellow, white, and kernels, on the cob
- ❖ Cucumber
- ❖ Cranberries
- ❖ Daikon
- ❖ Fresh Dates
- ❖ Shelled or pods Edamame

- ❖ Egg substitutes
- ❖ Dragon fruit
- ❖ Egg whites
- ❖ Eggplant
- ❖ Endive
- ❖ Whole Eggs with yolk
- ❖ Fennel (finocchio, anise or sweet anise)
- ❖ Figs
- ❖ Escarole
- ❖ Fish: sea bass, sardines, smoked lox, salmon, all varieties of salmon, sablefish, roe, steelhead rainbow trout, pompano, Pollack, pike, perch, orange roughy, monkfish, dolphinfish (mahimahi), mackerel, herring, halibut, haddock, grouper, gefilte fish, flounder, eel, drum, cod, catfish, carp, butterfish, sea bass (branzino), bluefish, arctic char and anchovies. Whitefish, pike, turbot, all varieties of tuna, tilefish, tilapia, swordfish, pumpkinseed (sunfish), white sucker, smoked sturgeon, striped mullet, striped bass, sole, snapper, smelt
- ❖ Grilled fish fillet with some lemon pepper
- ❖ Unsweetened Fruit cup
- ❖ Fruit salad
- ❖ Fruit cocktail
- ❖ Unsweetened fruit
- ❖ Ginger root
- ❖ Garlic
- ❖ Grapes
- ❖ Grapefruit
- ❖ Greens: dandelion, beet, and collard, kale, turnip and mustard,
- ❖ Mixed baby Greens
- ❖ Guavas and strawberry
- ❖ (Palmetto) Hearts of palm
- ❖ Canned Hominy
- ❖ Honeydew melon
- ❖ Chicken breast, Jerk

- ❖ Jackfruit
- ❖ Sunchokes (Jerusalem artichokes)
- ❖ Yam bean (Jicama)
- ❖ Kohlrabi
- ❖ Kiwifruit
- ❖ Kumquats
- ❖ Lemon
- ❖ Leeks
- ❖ Lemon zest
- ❖ All varieties of Lettuce
- ❖ Lentils
- ❖ Lime
- ❖ Lime zest
- ❖ Lychees (Litchis)
- ❖ Melon balls
- ❖ Mangoes
- ❖ Sprouts Mung bean
- ❖ Mushroom caps
- ❖ Mung Dal
- ❖ All varieties of Mushrooms like shiitake, portabella, Italian, Crimini, button and brown
- ❖ Nectarine
- ❖ Okra
- ❖ Nori seaweed
- ❖ Onions
- ❖ All varieties of Oranges like blood
- ❖ Parsley
- ❖ Papayas
- ❖ Passionfruit
- ❖ Peaches
- ❖ Pea Shoots
- ❖ Black-eye Peapods
- ❖ Pears

- ❖ Carrots and peas
- ❖ Peas: sugar snap, split, Chinese pods, pea snow, pigeon, green, pods young with seeds, cowpeas (southern, crowder and black eyes), black-eyed and garbanzo (chickpeas)
- ❖ All varieties of Peppers
- ❖ Persimmons
- ❖ Pepperoncini
- ❖ Unsweetened Pickles
- ❖ Canned Pimientos
- ❖ Pico de gallo
- ❖ Pluots (Plumcots)
- ❖ Pineapple
- ❖ Pomegranate seeds
- ❖ Plums
- ❖ Pomegranates
- ❖ Pummelo (Pomelo)
- ❖ Pumpkin puree
- ❖ Pumpkin
- ❖ Radicchio
- ❖ Raspberries
- ❖ Radishes
- ❖ Rutabagas
- ❖ Mixed green Salad
- ❖ Side salad without any dressing, fast food
- ❖ Three-bean Salad
- ❖ Tossed saladwithout dressing
- ❖ Fat-free Salsa
- ❖ Salsa verde
- ❖ Gluten-free and fat-free Salsa
- ❖ Chicken Satay without any peanut sauce
- ❖ Sashimi
- ❖ Sauerkraut
- ❖ Satsuma Mandarin

- ❖ Scallions
- ❖ Shallots
- ❖ Seaweed
- ❖ Shellfish: squid, shrimp, scallops, oysters, octopus, mussels, lobster, spiny lobster, cuttlefish, crayfish, crab (including queen, crabmeat lump, Dungeness, blue, king and Alaska), clams and abalone
- ❖ Spinach
- ❖ All varieties Squash, zucchini and summer
- ❖ Sprouts like lentils, alfalfa and bean
- ❖ All varieties of winter Squash like spaghetti
- ❖ Strawberries
- ❖ Starfruit (carambola)
- ❖ Succotash
- ❖ Tangerine
- ❖ Tangelo
- ❖ Taro
- ❖ All varieties of Tofu
- ❖ Smoked Tofu
- ❖ Tomato puree
- ❖ Tomatillos
- ❖ Tomato sauce
- ❖ All varieties of Tomatoes like cherry, plum, and grape
- ❖ Fat-free ground Turkey breast
- ❖ Tenderloin or Turkey breast boneless, skinless and with bone
- ❖ Turnips
- ❖ Smoked Turkey breast (skinless)
- ❖ Vegetables, mixed
- ❖ Vegetable sticks
- ❖ Stir fry vegetables without sauce
- ❖ Watercress
- ❖ Water chestnuts
- ❖ Watermelon
- ❖ Greek plain Yogurt, Greek (unsweetened and non-fat)

- ❖ Yogurt, plain ((unsweetened and non-fat)
- ❖ Soy Yogurt, plain

Credit of Food List: Weight Watchers International Inc.

Tips for Successful Weight Watchers Freestyle Program

If you want to increase the success of your Weight Watchers Freestyle program, you must strictly follow your daily allocation SmartPoints. Here are some tips for successful Weight Watchers Freestyle program:

Drink Plenty of Water

Water is an essential component of your diet. It plays a vital role in your success. Your body needs water throughout a day to operate appropriately. Dehydration can widely affect functions of your body. You have to focus on getting almost 65 ounces water on a daily basis.

Make an Eating Plan

Meal planning can increase the success chances of your weight watcher program. You must take one hour or even more to plan a meal for each week. You can include snacks in your diet. Prepare a grocery list as per your meal plan and stock your pantry with healthy items. Make sure to avoid a visit to the grocery store while you feel hungry.

Smart Substitute of Cravings

Hunger pangs are inevitable, especially when you have initially started a diet program. Weight Watchers freestyle recommends you to satisfy your cravings. For instance, if you want to eat sugar, you can satisfy your hunger by eating a fruit. If you need something crunchy and salty, try delicious popcorns instead of unhealthy chips.

Make Physical Activity a Fun

Exercise is not about lifting weight and running on a treadmill. You can try other fun options to sweat, such as swimming, cycling, yoga, and Pilates. It will be good to call your friends and plan a running or morning walk with them.

Bank up Extra Points for Delicious Treats

Weight Watchers Freestyle allow you to enjoy your favorite treats. You can rollover your SmartPoints to the next day budget of SmartPoints. On a weekday, when you have sufficient balance of extra points, you can consume something delicious and sweet like a chocolate cake or ice cream.

FAQs

Q: How WW Freestyle determines a zero point food?

A: Their zero point food category consists of lean protein, vegetables, and fruits. These food items offer a foundation that helps you to build healthy eating patterns. These food items provide top-quality nutrition that becomes the foundation of your healthy diet without increasing the risk of overindulgence. It is easy to avoid overeating because it is hard to eat six pieces of chicken than six chocolate cookies.

Q: What is the difference between WW Freestyle program and Filling Technique?

A: Freestyle allows members to roll over four unused regular SmartPoints in a day into weekly budget. With simple filling technique, the list of no-count food items is broader. The members of regular filling plan can't get flexibility dials other than their list. The main differences between these programs are as under:

➢ Freestyle offers a SmartPoints budget that contains weekly and daily SmartPoints. The simply filing offers only weekly SmartPoints.

➢ While following simply filling, you will get a broad list of "free" food items. The Freestyle offers a particular list of food with zero SmartPoints and particular bread, whole grains, cheese, yogurt, skim milk, lean cuts of meat and healthy oil (only two teaspoons).

➤ WW Freestyle makes it possible for you to accumulate almost four unused SmartPoints regularly to rollover extra points to your weekly budget. However, Simply Filling has no such facility.

Q: Why are peas and beans in the list of zero Points food? Peas and beans have a right amount of carbs?

A: As per latest dietary guidelines, healthy consumption includes lots of vegetables from five subgroups of vegetable, such as starchy, red, orange and dark green legumes (peas and beans). These foods have a right amount of fiber than other food items. These are nutritious and filling, so members of WW freestyle are encouraged to consume them.

Chapter 2 – Seven Day WW Freestyle meal plan

See this sample WW Freestyle meal plan. You can make some modifications in the meal plan as per your needs.

Sunday

Breakfast: 1 Quiche Serving, Yogurt Parfait
Lunch: 6 oz. chicken Parmesan, Cinnamon Muffin
Dinner: Chicken Meatballs, Grilled Shrimps

Monday

Breakfast: Scrambled eggs with veggies, 1 Yogurt Pancake,
Lunch: Chicken and Mushrooms, Applesauce Cookie,
Dinner: Chicken pasta, Chickpea Salad, Cinnamon Muffin

Tuesday

Breakfast: 1 Serving casserole, 1 oatmeal muffin
Lunch: Chicken Fajitas, Green Salad
Dinner: 2 Lasagna Rolls up, Chicken Verde, Ice Cream

Wednesday

Breakfast: 1 French Toast with cinnamon and Apple, Mint Fluff, Cinnamon Muffin
Lunch: 1 Fish Burger, 1/2 serving black bean and summer squash, Jello Cookie
Dinner: 2 Spinach Manicotti, 3 Chicken Nuggets, 1/2 serving Applesauce

Thursday

Breakfast: 1 Serving casserole, 1 oatmeal muffin
Lunch: Chicken Fajitas, 1 Fish burger, Green Salad
Dinner: 2 cups potato soup, Baked Salmon, 1 Baked Pear with honey and walnut

Friday

Breakfast: 1 French Toast with cinnamon and Apple
Lunch: Parmesan Shrimp with Garlic, 1 Fish Burger
Dinner: 3 ounces BBQ Apricot Chicken, Baked Mushrooms or Green Beans

Saturday

Breakfast: 1 Serving casserole, 1 oatmeal muffin
Lunch: Tuna Salad with cranberry, Chicken Fajita,
Dinner: Chicken Sautéed Rice, Tangy Chili, Ice Cream

Chapter 3 – WW Freestyle Breakfast Recipes

Start your day with a delicious breakfast. Here are some WW Freestyle breakfast recipes to make your morning healthy.

Recipe 01: Yummy Quiche Recipe

Freestyle Smart Points: 1, 1/4 Quiche
Total Time: 30 minutes
Servings: 4

Ingredients:

- 3 organic eggs
- 4 organic egg whites
- 5 quartered cherry tomatoes
- 2/3 cup chopped asparagus, chop into 1-inch pieces
- 1/3 cup chopped bell pepper, green
- 1/2 cup mozzarella cheese, shredded
- Pepper and salt to taste

Directions:

1) Whisk whole eggs and egg white in a bowl until smooth, keep aside.
2) Chop bell peppers, tomatoes, asparagus, and mix into whisked egg bowl.
3) Stir in only half of the parmesan cheese.
4) Use some olive oil to grease one pie dish and transfer egg mixture in this dish.
5) Top egg mixture with remaining cheese and bake at 350°F for almost 35 to 40 minutes.

Recipe 02: Healthy Egg Scramble with Vegetables

Freestyle Smart Points: 3
Total Time: 15 minutes
Servings: 6

Ingredients:

- 3 cups baby spinach, organic
- 6 organic large eggs
- 1/2 diced red onion, organic
- 1 organic diced tomato
- 1 clove minced and crushed garlic
- 1 teaspoon pink salt
- 1 teaspoon black pepper, cracked
- 1/2 cup cheddar cheese, organic
- 1-1/2 tablespoon olive oil, extra virgin

Directions:

1) Whisk eggs together in a bowl. Mix in salt and black pepper and keep aside.
2) Heat olive oil in a large pan. Ad in garlic, onion, spinach, tomato, and sauté for almost 5 to 7 minutes to cook veggies.
3) Pour whisked eggs over sautéed veggies and cook for extra 3 to 4 minutes. Stir occasionally and cook to set eggs.
4) Turn off heat and sprinkle eggs with some cheese. Serve hot.

Recipe 03: Yogurt Parfait

Freestyle Smart Points: 1
Total Time: 10 minutes
Servings: 1

Ingredients:

- 1 cup Greek Yogurt, non-fat
- 1 packet Splenda
- 1/2 teaspoon organic vanilla extract
- 8 pretzels of any brand
- 10 chopped strawberries

Directions:

1) Put all pretzels in a plastic zip bag and use a mallet to smash them.
2) Layer the yogurt, pretzels and strawberries. You can make 2 to 3 layers. Serve.

Recipe 04: Yogurt Pancakes

Freestyle Smart Points: 1 for each pancake
Total Time: 20 minutes
Servings: 14

Ingredients:

- 1 cup all-purpose flour
- 2 cups plain Greek yogurt, nonfat
- 2 teaspoons baking soda
- 4 whisked eggs
- 1 teaspoon salt
- 1/2 cup low-fat 1% milk
- 1 teaspoon vanilla

Directions:

1) Take a medium mixing bowl and pour yogurt into this bowl. Combine remaining dry ingredients and mix into yogurt. Stir well until dry ingredients are completely incorporated in the yogurt.
2) Combine vanilla, milk, and eggs. Add this blend to yogurt blend and mix well to combine.
3) Grease a griddle pan or skillet and pour 1/2-cup batter to make a pancake of 5-inch diameter. Cook for 2 minutes to make its one side golden brown. Now flip this pancake when bubbles appear on the uncooked side. Cook this side for 1 to 2 minutes until golden brown.
4) Replicate this procedure with remaining batter to make almost 14 pancakes. Serve hot with your favorite syrup.

Recipe 05: Yummy Breakfast Casserole

Freestyle Smart Points: 1 for 1/4 section of casserole
Total Time: 30 minutes
Servings: 4

Ingredients:

- 1/4 cup shredded cheddar cheese, fat free
- 6 organic eggs
- 4 chopped turkey sausages
- 1/4 cup chopped cherry tomatoes
- 1/2 chopped red onion
- 1/2 red or green bell pepper
- 1/4 cup chopped mushrooms
- Garlic salt, to taste
- Pepper, to taste
- Red pepper flakes, to taste
- Oregano, to taste

Directions:

1) Crack eggs in one bowl and whisk well.
2) Add cheese, sausages, cherry tomatoes, red onion, bell pepper, mushrooms, garlic salt, pepper, red pepper flakes and oregano in whisked eggs.
3) Mix well and transfer this blend to a greased casserole dish.
4) Bake this blend for almost 35 minutes at 350°F or until cooked through. Serve hot.

Recipe 06: Mouthwatering Oatmeal Muffins

Freestyle Smart Points: 2 in 1 muffin
Total Time: 40 minutes
Servings: 12

Ingredients:

- 1 egg
- 2 mashed bananas, medium
- 1 teaspoon vanilla
- 1/3 cup skim milk
- 1 teaspoon baking powder
- 2-1/4 cup large flake Quaker oats
- 1/2 teaspoon cinnamon
- Raspberry, apricot or mixed fruit jam without sugar

Directions:

1) Preheat your oven to 350°F. Spray 12 muffin tins with non-stick cooking spray.
2) Whisk egg and milk together in a bowl. Mix in vanilla and mashed banana.
3) Mix in cinnamon, baking powder, and oats.
4) Divide batter between 12 greased muffin cups. Make an indent in the center of each muffin to add jam. Drop 1/2 to 1 tablespoon of jam in each muffin.
5) Bake for almost 22 minutes in your preheated oven.
6) You can store these muffins in the fridge for a few days.

Recipe 07: French Toast with Cinnamon and Apple

Freestyle Smart Points: 6 for each toast
Total Time: 55 minutes
Servings: 4

Ingredients:

- 2 diced and peeled apples
- 8 medium-sized slices of brown bread
- 4 eggs
- 2 teaspoons cinnamon
- 1 1/3 cup egg whites
- 1 cup milk, 1%

Directions:

1) Preheat your oven to exactly 350°F. Spray one casserole dish (9x13) with non-stick cooking spray.
2) Mix 1-teaspoon cinnamon and diced apples in a bowl (microwave safe). Cover this bowl tightly with saran wrap and put in the microwave for almost 3 minutes. Stir well.
3) Spread four slices of bread in a dish and equally top all slices with apples. Put remaining four slices over apples to make healthy sandwiches.
4) Take a bowl to whisk egg whites and egg together. Mix in milk and 1-teaspoon cinnamon. Pour this mixture over bread sandwiches to cover them well. The mixture can spread in the dish, but don't worry because it will be the part of serving.
5) Bake sandwiches in oven for almost 45 minutes to cook eggs.
6) Serve with sugar-free syrup. Keep it in mind that two tablespoons of syrup will be equal to 1 smart freestyle points.

Recipe 08: Kale and Bacon Salad

Freestyle Smart Points: 4
Total Time: 15 minutes
Servings: 2

Ingredients:

- 3 cups kale, shredded without stems
- 1 teaspoon vinegar, red wine
- 2 teaspoons olive oil, extra virgin
- Pink salt, to taste
- 2 eggs
- Ground black pepper, as per taste
- 4 strips chopped cooked bacon, center cut
- 10 tomatoes, halved
- 2 ounces avocado, sliced

Direction:

1) Combine salt (1/4 teaspoon), vinegar, olive oil and kale in one bowl. Mix with your hands for almost 3 minutes.
2) Boil eggs (as per desired likeness) soft or hard.
3) Divide kale between serving bowls. Top with avocado, egg, tomatoes, and bacon. Season with pepper and salt. Serve.

Recipe 09: Appetizing Baked Taquitos

Freestyle Smart Points: 2 for each taquito
Total Time: 30 minutes
Servings: 5

Ingredients:

- 10 (6-inch) corn tortillas
- 1 finely chopped bell pepper, red
- 3 scrambled eggs
- 1/2 cup spinach, chopped
- 1 thinly sliced green onion
- 1 to 2 tablespoons jalapeno, minced

Direction:

1) Preheat your oven to almost 425°F.
2) Take one baking dish and spray it with your nonstick spray. Keep it aside.
3) Scramble eggs in a pan as per your taste.
4) Microwave corn tortillas for almost 1 minutes to make them soft.
5) Take a bowl and mix remaining ingredients and scrambled eggs to make a delicious filling.
6) Spoon almost one tablespoon over one heated corn tortilla.
7) Carefully wrap this tortilla upward around the filling. Wrap all tortillas.
8) Put the seam area down on the greased baking dish. Arrange all tortillas in the baking dish and bake for almost 12 to 15 minutes to make them crispy. Serve hot.

Recipe 10: Scrambled Egg

Freestyle Smart Points: 2
Total Time: 15 minutes
Servings: 2

Ingredients:

- 1 tablespoon melted butter
- 1/2 cup feta cheese, crumbled
- Pepper and salt, to taste
- 3 eggs
- 1 teaspoon fresh water

Direction:

1) Take a pan and heat butter in this pan over medium flame.
2) Whisk water and eggs together and pour in the pan. Stir in feta cheese and occasionally stir for scrambling.
3) Season with pepper and salt. Serve.

Recipe 11: Cauliflower Rice

Freestyle Smart Points: 1 for 1 cup serving
Total Time: 10 minutes
Servings: 1

Ingredients:

- 4 cups crumbles cauliflower
- 1 teaspoon coconut or olive oil
- 2 plum medium tomatoes, diced
- 1/2 finely diced onion, medium
- 2 minced garlic cloves
- 1 minced jalapeno, membrane and seeds removed
- 2 tablespoons fresh tomato paste
- 1/4 paprika, smoked
- 1/2 teaspoon roasted cumin
- 1 teaspoon pink salt
- 1/4 teaspoon ground cayenne pepper
- Chopped cilantro
- Ground black pepper, as per taste

Direction:

1) Take a large pan and heat oil in it over medium heat. Add jalapeno, tomatoes, and onion in hot oil and sauté for almost 2 to 3 minutes. Mix in cauliflower and garlic, sauté cauliflower for nearly 2 minutes.
2) Mix in pepper, salt, cayenne, paprika, cumin and tomato paste. Mix to equally coat vegetables. Cook for almost 1 minutes to heat through. Mix in chopped cilantro. Serve hot.

Recipe 12: Oatmeal Pancakes

Freestyle Smart Points: 6 (2 pancakes in one serving)
Total Time: 15 minutes
Servings: 4

Ingredients:

- 1/2 cup cottage cheese, low fat
- 1 cup oats, old fashioned
- 2 teaspoon vanilla extract
- 8 organic egg whites
- 1/2 teaspoon pumpkin pie spice
- 1/2 teaspoon cinnamon

Direction:

1) Use a regular blender or immersion blender to combine all ingredients to make a smooth batter.
2) Use one quarter cup to pour batter into one heated pan greased with olive oil. Flip pancake once the top starts to pop and bubble.
3) Cook for 1 to 2 minutes. Serve with maple syrup or honey and fruits.
4) Note: If you want sweet pancakes, you can add some brown sugar, honey or stevia in pancake batter.

Chapter 4 – WW Freestyle Lunch Recipes

A healthy lunch is necessary to increase your energy. Energize your body with these yummy and healthy lunch recipes.

Recipe 01: Delicious Chicken Parmesan

Freestyle Smart Points: 5 in 6 oz. chicken
Total Time: 30 minutes
Servings: 4

Ingredients:

- 1 pound skinless and boneless chicken cutlets
- 1/4 cup breadcrumbs, panko
- 1 whisked egg
- 1/4 cup parmesan cheese, grated
- 1 teaspoon Italian seasoning
- 1 teaspoon garlic powder
- Pepper and salt, as per taste
- 2 teaspoons olive oil
- 3 cups fresh green beans
- 1/2 cup spicy marinara sauce
- 1/4 cup chopped fresh basil
- 1/2 cup mozzarella cheese, shredded

Directions:

1) Preheat your oven to 425°F. Use a non-stick cooking spray to spray your baking sheet or use a foil to cover for easy cleanup.

2) Combine pepper, salt, Italian seasoning, garlic powder, parmesan cheese, and panko breadcrumbs in a bowl.

3) Press a side of chicken in the whisked egg and the parmesan and panko mixture. Put this chicken slice over a baking sheet with breading up. Replicate this process with remaining slices of chicken. If you want to increase the crispy texture of chicken, spray it with some olive oil.

4) Toss green beans with olive oil and sprinkle some pepper and salt as per taste. Spread out these beans around chicken over a baking sheet.

5) Cook for almost 15 minutes in your preheated oven to tender chicken. Remove pan from oven and top each chicken piece with mozzarella cheese and marinara sauce. Return this baking dish in the oven to cook for 1 to 2 minutes.

6) Top with basil or mint and serve hot.

Recipe 02: Mouthwatering Chicken with Mushrooms

Freestyle Smart Points: 1 for 1/2 cup mushrooms & 6 oz. chicken
Total Time: 25 minutes
Servings: 4

Ingredients:

- 1.33 pounds skinless and boneless chicken breast
- 8 oz. sliced mushrooms
- 2 teaspoons olive oil
- 2 minced garlic cloves
- 1/2 cup chicken broth, low-sodium
- 1-1/2 tablespoons balsamic vinegar
- Pepper and salt, to taste
- 1 tablespoon chopped parsley
- 1/2 teaspoon thyme

Directions:

1) Use pepper and salt to season chicken. Heat olive oil in a pan over medium heat. Add chicken in hot oil and carefully sear both sides of chicken for 2 to 3 minutes, until light brown. Remove chicken and keep aside.
2) Now add mushrooms and garlic to skillet and cook for 3 to 4 minutes to tender mushrooms.
3) Add thyme, balsamic vinegar, and chicken broth to your skillet. Mix and scrape browned chicken bits off the base of the skillet. Add chicken and simmer it for almost 10 to 15 minutes over low heat, until thoroughly cooked.

Recipe 03: Chicken Fajitas

Freestyle Smart Points: 1 for 1 cup
Total Time: 40 minutes
Servings: 4

Ingredients:

- 1.33 lbs skinless and boneless chicken breast, chop into strips
- 1 sliced onion
- 14 ounces diced tomatoes and green chiles
- 1 sliced red pepper
- 1 sliced green pepper
- 2 teaspoons vegetable oil
- 1 cup sliced mushrooms
- 1-1/2 teaspoon cumin
- 1-1/2 teaspoon chili powder
- 1 teaspoon paprika
- 1/2 teaspoon onion powder
- 1/2 teaspoon garlic powder
- 1/2 teaspoon dried oregano
- 1/4 teaspoon salt

Directions:

1) Preheat your oven to precisely 400°F.
2) Add each ingredient in a baking dish (glass dish) and toss everything with your hands. For your convenience, you can add chicken, veggies, and tomatoes. Sprinkle oil and spices on top and toss.
3) Bake for almost 25 to 30 minutes until cook through. Serve hot.

Recipe 04: Mouthwatering Fish Burgers

Freestyle Smart Points: 5 in 1 burger
Total Time: 20 minutes
Servings: 4

Ingredients:

- 1/4 cup Panko seasoned breadcrumbs
- 1 pound tilapia
- 1 egg white
- 1 egg
- 2 tablespoons Dijon Mustard
- 1 minced garlic clove
- 1 teaspoon salt
- 1 teaspoon onion powder
- 1/2 teaspoon black pepper
- 1 teaspoon paprika
- 1 teaspoon vegetable oil
- 1/2 teaspoon basil
- 4 hamburger buns, reduced calorie
- 1 sliced tomato
- I sliced cucumber
- 1/2 avocado

Directions:

1) Put fish in your food processor and pulse it to chop.
2) Combine chopped fish with egg white, egg, breadcrumbs, onion powder, basil, paprika, pepper, salt, garlic, and mustard.
3) Put this blend in a fridge for almost 10 minutes before making patties. After 10 minutes, form patties with this blend.
4) Brush all burgers with olive oil.
5) Grease a skillet and cook patties in this skillet over medium flame for almost 4 minutes each side.
6) Serve patties on toasted burger buns with tomato slices and avocado.

_e 05: Tasty Parmesan Shrimps with Garlic

Freestyle Smart Points: 4 for 6 oz.
Total Time: 15 minutes
Servings: 4

Ingredients:

- 2 tablespoons olive oil or melted butter
- 1.33 lbs deveined, peeled and raw shrimp
- 3 minced garlic cloves
- 1/4 cup grated parmesan
- 1 teaspoon Italian seasoning
- 1 lime or lemon juice
- Pepper and salt, to taste

Directions:

1) Preheat your oven to precisely 300°F.
2) Toss all shrimps with parmesan cheese, Italian seasoning, garlic, and olive oil. Put tossed shrimps in one layer on your baking sheet.
3) Cook in your preheated oven for almost 6 to 8 minutes to cook through. Serve with lemon juice.

Recipe 06: Appetizing Tuna Salad with Cranberry

Freestyle Smart Points: 3 for 2/3 cup
Total Time: 10 minutes
Servings: 5

Ingredients:

- 3 tablespoons low-fat mayonnaise
- 16 ounces white tuna, water packed, drained
- 3 tablespoons sour cream, light
- 1/2 cup chopped celery
- 1/4 cup minced red onion
- 1/4 cup cranberries, dried
- 1 tablespoons lemon juice
- 1 diced apple
- Pepper and salt, to taste

Directions:

1) Take a bowl and combine mayonnaise, white tuna, sour cream, celery, red onion, cranberries, lemon juice, apple, salt, and pepper in this bowl.
2) Mix well and put in the fridge to serve chilled. You can eat right away.

Recipe 07: Tangy Black Beans and Summer Squash

Freestyle Smart Points: 3 for 2 squash halves
Total Time: 50 minutes
Servings: 4

Ingredients:

- 2 cups black beans, drained and rinsed
- 4 zucchini or summer squash
- 1 minced garlic clove
- 1 cup minced onion
- 1/2 cup diced bell pepper, red
- 1/2 teaspoon cumin
- 1/2 cup shredded reduced fat cheddar cheese
- 1 cup red enchilada sauce

Directions:

1) Preheat your oven to precisely 400°F.
2) Take summer squash and scoop out its middle. Chop the scooped out squash to make it a part of your filling.
3) Put a skillet over medium heat and add onion, scooped out pieces of squash, bell pepper, garlic and black beans in the skillet. Cook for almost 5 to 7 minutes to tender.
4) Stir in pepper, salt, and cumin. Add enchilada sauce to the mixture.
5) Fill every summer squash with this blend and put in the baking dish. Sprinkle each squash with cheese.
6) Cover the baking dish with a foil and put in a preheated oven to bake for almost 25 minutes. After this time, remove foil and bake again for 10 minutes.

Recipe 08: Tuna Salad

Freestyle Smart Points: 5 per serving
Total Time: 25 minutes
Servings: 6

Ingredients:

- 12 ounces tuna (can in water), drained
- 6 ounces pasta
- 1/2 cup halved cherry tomato
- 1/2 cup bell pepper, yellow (chop into strips)
- 1/4 cup diced celery
- 3/4 cup salsa, low-salt
- 1/2 cup mayonnaise, low-fat
- 1/2 teaspoon red pepper, ground
- 2 tablespoons sliced scallion

Direction:

1) Cook pasta per package directions, omit fat and salt.
2) Drain pasta and rinse under chilled water. Drain and keep aside.
3) Combine celery, cherry tomatoes, bell pepper, tuna and pasta in a bowl.
4) Take another bowl and combine red pepper, mayonnaise, and salsa. Add this dressing to pasta mixture. Toss well, cover and put in the fridge.
5) Sprinkle some scallions over pasta before serving.

Recipe 09: Turkey Chili

Freestyle Smart Points: 6
Total Time: 1 hour 20 minutes
Servings: 8

Ingredients:

- 1/2 cup onion, diced
- 1/4 teaspoon black pepper, ground
- 1/4 teaspoon dry oregano
- 1/2 teaspoon pink salt
- 1 teaspoon cumin, ground
- 1/4 teaspoon ground cayenne pepper
- 2 can white beans (15 to 16 oz)
- 2 cups chicken broth
- 1 tablespoons garlic, minced
- 2 tablespoons coconut or olive oil
- 1/2 cup celery, diced
- 1/2 diced green pepper
- 2 cups cooked turkey, shredded
- Parmesan cheese, shredded for topping
- Cilantro and sour cream for serving

Direction:

1) Take a Dutch oven or stockpot. Add olive oil, celery, green pepper and onion in the pot. Cook over medium heat to tender peppers and make onion translucent. Mix in garlic.
2) Add turkey, beans, and chicken broth and stir well. Mix in seasoning. Cook on high heat to boil and then decrease heat to cook for 30 to 60 minutes, stir occasionally.
3) Serve with cilantro, cheese, and sour cream.

Recipe 10: Tortillas Scrambled Eggs

Freestyle Smart Points: 5
Total Time: 20 minutes
Servings: 4

Ingredients:

- 4 tortillas – whole wheat flour
- 3 chopped shallots – Green
- 2 tablespoons milk – low fat
- 1 teaspoon red chili - chopped
- 5 eggs
- 60 g cheese – low fat
- 2 tablespoons coriander - chopped

Direction:

1) Follow the instruction on the packet of tortillas to warm them.
2) Great a non-stick pan with extra virgin olive oil and cook chili and shallots to cook on medium heat for 2 minutes.
3) Now whisk eggs with milk and sprinkle spices to taste. Now cook it in the pan on medium heat for 3 minutes and keep the tortillas on the serving plates. Cover tortilla with eggs, coriander and cheese. Roll up tortilla to serve.

Recipe 11: Apricot Cake in Crockpot

Freestyle Smart Points: 4
Total Time: 3 hours 30 minutes
Servings: 6

Ingredients:

- 1 teaspoon vanilla
- 3/4 cup sugar
- 1 large egg
- 1/4 cup crushed nuts.
- 3 tablespoons canola oil
- 1 cup all-purpose flour
- 1/4 teaspoon salt
- 1/2 teaspoon baking powder
- 1/2 teaspoon baking soda
- 2 cups chopped apricot

Directions:

1) In the first step, take a baking dish and grease it to fit in the slow cooker. You need a metal mason jar to place in the bottom of the slow cooker to offer support to the pan.
2) Take a medium bowl and beat sugar, egg, vanilla and oil to get a blended cream. Mix flour into this mixture and add apricot as well as walnuts. Take a separate bowl and beat baking soda, flour, baking powder, and salt.
3) Scuff the batter equally into the greased pan and use a foil to cover this pan. Adjust in the slow cooker and cover the lid to bake on high setting for 2 to 3 hours. You can use a toothpick to check the cake, insert it in the center and check if it comes out clean. You can cover the cake for more 15 to 30 minutes, if it is not done.
4) After baking the cake, take it out from the cooker and keep it on the rack to cool for almost 15 to 20 minutes. Cut into 8 slices and serve.

Recipe 12: Apple and Potato Tart

Freestyle Smart Points: 5
Total Time: 1 hour
Servings: 4

Ingredients:

- 4 chopped potatoes
- 1 chopped apple
- 1 chopped onion
- 2 tablespoons chopped parsley
- 1/2 teaspoon salt
- 2 tablespoons olive oil
- 1/2 cup grated cheese – gruyere

Directions:

1) Heat an oven at almost 425 degrees Fahrenheit and grease a baking pan with edible olive oil. Now add potatoes, apple, onion, olive oil, parsley, pepper and salt in a large brown and mix them well.
2) Now pour half of this mixture in the baking pan and sprinkle a 1/4th cup of cheese. Now pour remaining half of the cheese layer and cover the cake with a greased aluminum foil to maintain moisture.
3) Bake for 40 minutes, then remove foil, and sprinkle ¼ cup of remaining cheese. Bake it for another 15 minutes and cut into equal slices to enjoy.

Chapter 5 – WW Freestyle Dinner Recipes

Make your dinner special with these delicious and tangy recipes. Here are some great options for your WW freestyle diet.

Recipe 01: Flavorful Chicken Meatballs

Freestyle Smart Points: 5 for 5 meatballs with mushrooms
Total Time: 30 minutes
Servings: 5

Ingredients:

- 1 pound ground chicken, lean
- 8 ounces cremini mushrooms, sliced and divided
- 1/3 cup seasoned whole wheat bread crumbs
- 1/4 cup Pecorino grated cheese
- 1 beaten large egg
- 3 garlic minced cloves
- 2 tablespoons fresh chopped parsley + extra for garnish
- 1 teaspoon Pink salt
- 1/2 tablespoon wheat or all-purpose flour
- Ground black pepper, to taste
- 1/2 tablespoon butter, unsalted
- 1/4 cup chopped shallots, finely chopped
- 3 ounces shiitake mushrooms, sliced
- 3/4 cup chicken broth, reduced sodium
- 1/3 cup red or Marsala wine

Directions:

1) Preheat your oven to almost 400°F.
2) Take a bowl and add chopped Cremini mushrooms, breadcrumbs, ground chicken, egg, Pecorino, minced garlic (1 clove) and parsley, black pepper, and 1 teaspoon salt in this bowl.
3) Mix well and gently shape this blend into 25 meatballs. Bake these meatballs on a greased baking pan for almost 15 – 18 minutes to make them golden.
4) Take a separate bowl and whisk in wine, broth, and flour.
5) Heat a skillet over medium flame. Add shallots, garlic, and butter in the skillet and cook for almost 2 minutes to make them golden and soft.
6) Stir in mushrooms and add one pinch of ground black pepper and salt (1/8 teaspoon). Cook for almost 5 minutes until golden. Stir occasionally.
7) Return baked meatballs to a pot and pour wine mixture over meatballs. Cover and cook for almost 10 minutes. Use parsley to garnish.

Recipe 02: Palatable Chicken Pasta

Freestyle Smart Points: 7 for 1 ½ cups
Total Time: 40 minutes
Servings: 8

Ingredients:

- 12 ounces penne pasta
- 2 cups cubed or shredded chicken
- 8 ounces cream cheese, fat-free
- 1/2 cup hot sauce
- 1/2 cup sour cream, fat-free
- 1 ounce ranch seasoning blend
- 1 cup cheddar cheese, fat-free and divided

Directions:

1) Preheat your oven to precisely 375°F.
2) Cook pasta as per the instructions on the package, drain and keep aside.
3) Grease a casserole dish with a nonstick spray.
4) Take a bowl and mix cheese (1/2 cup), sour cream, ranch mix, hot sauce, cream cheese and chicken in this bowl. Stir in drained pasta.
5) Pour this blend in a casserole dish and equally spread this mixture.
6) Top it with remaining fat-free cheese and bake for almost 18 to 20 minutes to melt cheese and heat through. Serve hot.

Recipe 03: Yummy Lasagna Roll Ups

Freestyle Smart Points: 7 for 2 rolls
Total Time: 40 minutes
Servings: 4

Ingredients:

- 15 ounces tomato sauce
- 8 raw lasagna noodles
- 1/2 teaspoon tangy Italian seasoning
- 1 cup thick pizza sauce
- 1 pounds raw poultry Italian sausage, remove casing (you can choose turkey or chicken sausage)
- 15 ounces ricotta cheese, fat-free
- 10 ounces chopped spinach
- 2 ounces chopped turkey pepperoni (reserve 8 un-chopped slices to use as topping)
- 2 ounces shredded mozzarella cheese
- 1 large egg

Directions:

1) Preheat your oven to precisely 350°F. Lightly grease a baking dish (9x13) with olive oil and keep aside.
2) Fill a pot with water and mix some salt in it. Boil this water to cook lasagna noodles as per the instructions to package. Rinse and drain with chilled water. Spread noodles flat on a dry and clean surface. Keep aside.
3) Combine Italian seasoning, pizza sauce and tomato sauce in a bowl. Stir together and put aside.
4) Put the chopped sausages in a skillet over medium heat and cook for a few minutes until browned. Break the meat into small pieces while

cooking. After cooking sausages, add 1/3 cup tomato sauce blend and chopped pepperoni. Mix well to combine. Turn off heat.

5) Combine egg, spinach and ricotta cheese in a bowl and mix well. Spoon almost 1/3 cup of cheese blend on every lasagna noodle and spread this blend crossways the surface. Make sure to leave the nearly 1/2-inch room without toppings. Top each cheese layer over noodles with meat mixture. Equally divide meat between noodles. Roll each noodle one by one over filling until it turns into a roll. Replicate this procedure with all noodles.

6) Spread 1/2 cup of tomato sauce blend in the bottom of your greased baking dish. Put lasagna rolls over tomato sauce (put each seam down) and pour remaining sauce over noodles. Top each roll with mozzarella cheese and put pepperoni on every noodle. Cover this dish with an aluminum foil and put in the oven for almost 40 minutes.

Recipe 04: Yummy Spinach Manicotti

Freestyle Smart Points: 7 for 2 manicotti
Total Time: 30 minutes
Servings: 8

Ingredients:

- 15 ounces ricotta cheese, skim
- 16 crespelles, homemade (see bonus recipes)
- 1 organic large egg
- 2 cups mozzarella cheese, shredded (reserve half cup)
- 10 ounces fresh peas
- 1/2 teaspoon pink salt
- 1/4 cup parmesan regianno, grated
- 2-1/2 cups marinara sauce (see bonus recipes)
- Black pepper, as per taste

Directions:

1) Make crespelles.
2) Preheat your oven to precisely 375°F.
3) Take a bowl and combine 1-1/2 cups of mozzarella, ricotta, spinach, egg, parmesan cheese, pepper and salt (1/2 teaspoon) in this bowl.
4) Fill every crespelle with spinach filling (almost 1/4 cup) and roll.
5) Take a baking dish (you can take two as per your need) and pour 1 cup sauce on its base. Put manicotti rolled (seem area down) on the baking dish. Top with remaining mozzarella cheese and 1-1/2 cups sauce.
6) Cover this dish with a foil and bake for almost 25 minutes, until bubbling and hot. Let the cheese melt. Serve hot.

Recipe 05: Appetizing Potato Soup

Freestyle Smart Points: 5 for 2 cups
Total Time: 45 minutes
Servings: 10

Ingredients:

- 1 diced carrot
- 2 cups cubed potatoes
- 2 thinly sliced leeks
- tablespoon extra-virgin olive oil
- 1 diced onion
- 4 cups chicken or vegetable broth
- 2 cups pure rice milk
- 2 cups fresh water
- 1/2 cup potato flakes
- 3 minced garlic cloves
- 2 tablespoons butter
- 2 tablespoons ground black pepper
- 2 tablespoons salt
- 1 teaspoon fine garlic powder
- 1 teaspoon fine onion powder
- 1 teaspoon paprika, smoked

Directions:

1) Take a stockpot (6-quart) and put on high heat. Add olive oil, garlic, carrots, leeks, and onions in the crockpot. Cook for almost 5 minutes, stir regularly to tender vegetables.
2) Mix in potatoes, milk, water, and broth. Let this mixture boil
3) Decrease heat to medium, add potatoes flakes, seasonings, and butter in the crockpot.
4) Continue cooking for almost 20 to 25 minutes, stir occasionally.
5) Taste to adjust seasoning as per your desire.
6) Serve potato soup with green onions, bacon, and dairy-free shredded cheese.

Recipe 06: Apricot BBQ Chicken

Freestyle Smart Points: 3 for 3 ounces serving
Total Time: 35 minutes
Servings: 6

Ingredients:

- 1/2 cup apricot jam, sugar-free
- pound skinless and boneless chicken breasts
- 1/2 cup BBQ Sauce, sugar-free
- 1 teaspoon ginger powder
- 1 teaspoon dry onion powder
- 1 teaspoon dry garlic powder
- 2 tablespoons soy sauce, low sodium

Directions:

1) Take a bowl and mix the seasonings, soy sauce, BBQ sauce and jam together.
2) Use a foil to line one baking sheet and put chicken breasts over foil in the equal layer.
3) Now pour BBQ sauce over meat to cover each piece of chicken.
4) Bake at 350°F for almost 30 minutes.
5) Take out the chicken and serve with salad.

Recipe 07: Delightful Chicken Sautéed Rice

Freestyle Smart Points: 2 for 1 cup
Total Time: 28 minutes
Servings: 6

Ingredients:

- 4 egg whites
- Cooking spray
- 1/2 cup raw chopped scallion, white and green parts
- 12 ounces raw skinless and boneless chicken breast, chop into cubes
- 2 cloves minced garlic cloves
- 1/2 cup diced uncooked carrots
- 2 cups regular long-grain brown rice, cooked
- 3 tablespoons soy sauce, low sodium
- 1/2 cup green peas

Directions:

1) Coat a nonstick pan with sufficient cooking spray. Put this pan over medium heat. Add whisked egg whites and cook well to scramble for almost 3 – 5 minutes. Stir frequently, remove from pan and keep aside.
2) Turn off heat, coat skillet again with sufficient cooking spray and put again over medium flame. Add garlic and scallions and sauté for two minutes. Add carrots and chicken, sauté to make chicken golden brown. Cook for almost 5 minutes.
3) Mix in scrambled egg whites, peas, soy sauce and brown rice (cooked). Stir twice for almost 1 minute. Serve hot.

Recipe 08: Beef Stew

Freestyle Smart Points: 3 (1 cup serving)
Total Time: 40 minutes
Servings: 8

Ingredients:

- Pepper and salt, to taste
- 1 lb beef cubes, lean
- 1 teaspoon coconut or olive oil
- 3 cups low-sodium beef broth
- 1 dry bay leaf
- 1/2 teaspoon dried oregano
- 2 minced garlic cloves
- 15 ounces tomato sauce
- 1 chopped onion, medium
- 1 cup chopped carrots
- 1 cup chopped celery
- 1 cup fresh or frozen corn
- 1.5 cups cubed red potatoes

Direction:

1) Click sauté on your Instant Pot. Add meat, dried oregano, onions, garlic, and olive oil. Cook meat for almost 4 minutes.
2) Add pepper, salt, celery, and carrots and sauté for almost 4 – 5 minutes.
3) Turn off its "Sauté" function and add remaining ingredients into your instant pot.
4) Hit "Manual button" and set time for 17 minutes or more as per the setting of your crockpot to tender meat.

Recipe 09: Bok Choy Salad

Freestyle Smart Points: 3
Total Time: 15 minutes
Servings: 2

Ingredients:

- 4 cups Bok Choy (finely chopped)
- 4 red onions (finely diced)
- 1/3 cup cilantro, (properly chopped)
- 2 tablespoon sesame oil
- 1 garlic clove, crushed
- 1/3 cup soy sauce
- 1 tablespoon vinegar (made of rice)
- 1 lime (Juice)
- 1 tablespoon honey
- 1-1/2 teaspoon fresh shredded ginger
- Pinch of red pepper peels

Directions:

1) Mix cabbage, onion, and cilantro in a bowl, while the remaining ingredients will be mixed in another bowl.
2) Pour this dressing with the cabbage and onion and leave it for 10 minutes. Shower the sesame seeds to enhance the flavor.

Recipe 10: Chicken Cacciatore in Slow Cooker

Freestyle Smart Points: 5
Total Time: 7 hours 10 minutes
Servings: 3

Ingredients:

- 1 Kg boneless, skinless chicken thighs/ breasts
- 3-4 pieces of garlic, crushed
- 2 to 3 spoons, chopped tomatoes
- 1/2 red chili, sliced in small pieces
- 1/2 Green chili, thinly sliced
- 1 onion, chopped
- 1 tablespoon of dried oregano
- 1 tablespoon basil
- 1 tablespoon salt/ according to the taste
- 1/2 tablespoon black pepper
- 1 leaf of bay
- 1/4 cups of water
- 1 packet of cooked pasta

Directions

1) Season chicken with salt and black pepper. Now add all the other ingredients and spices.
2) Mix well to combine all ingredients. Cover the crockpot, turn it on, and set it to slow for 7 hours to cook the chicken at low temperature.
3) Take out chicken, shred it and serve with pasta.

Recipe 11: Porcupine Balls in Crockpot

Freestyle Smart Points: 7
Total Time: 6 hours
Servings: 4

Ingredients:

- 1 pound ground Lamb
- 1 egg
- 1 can vegetable soup
- 2 tablespoons onion flakes, dry
- 1/4 teaspoon garlic powder
- Salt and pepper as per your taste
- 1/2 cup rice, cooked

Directions:

1) Take a bowl and mix ground meat, egg, salt, rice, and pepper. Prepare almost 16 balls of this mixture and place in the slow cooker in a single layer. Now add soup and cover the cooker on low setting for almost 4 to 6 hours.
2) Now adjust the meatballs in the single layer in a dish and pour in the soup. Bake it in a preheated oven in a 350 degree for almost 1 hour. The meatballs will be cooked properly and the sauce becomes bubbly.

Recipe 12: Cauliflower and Ginger Mash in Crockpot

Freestyle Smart Points: 4
Total Time: 2 hours
Servings: 8

Ingredients:

- Olive oil, 1 tablespoon
- Chicken Broth, 1/2 cup without salt
- 5 Ginger Pieces, chopped 1 tablespoon
- Plain yogurt, 1 cup
- Low-fat cream, 1/2 cup
- Salt as per taste
- 3 lbs cauliflower

Directions

1) Wash your cauliflower and chop it after removing its hard parts. Bake the cauliflower in the microwave for 15 minutes.
2) Remove them from the oven after they completely cooked. Cook garlic in the olive oil for 2 to 3 minutes.
3) Put cauliflower in the slow cooker with broth. Keep the ginger on the top and mix everything well.
4) Cook on a low setting for 1.5 hours, then place the pot on the heat-safe surface. You need a hand blender to mash the potato together with the yogurt and milk. Add salt as per your taste.

Chapter 6 – WW Freestyle Snack Recipes

You will need snacks to satisfy your hunger between meals. You can try these healthy snacks during meals.

Recipe 01: Tangy Chili

Freestyle Smart Points: 0, 1 1/3 cup serving
Total Time: 40 minutes
Servings: 10

Ingredients:

- 30 ounces kidney beans (rinsed and drained)
- 30 ounces pinto beans (rinsed and drained)
- 30 ounces black beans (rinsed and drained)
- 1 pound lean ground chicken
- 30 ounces Diced Tomatoes and Green Chilies
- 1/2 tablespoon oregano
- 1/2 tablespoon cumin
- 1 tablespoon chili powder
- 2 to 3 minced garlic cloves
- 1 diced onion
- 1 quartered lime
- 15 ounces tomato sauce

Directions:

1) Put ground meat in instant pot, use brown or sauté function to cook meat.

2) Pour remaining ingredients into instant pot other than lime. Quarter one lime and gently squeeze its juice in the pot. Throw the skin away.
3) Choose Meat/Stew or Beans/Chili button on the instant pot. Start your pot and carefully close it pressure valve. You have to cook for almost 20 to 35 minutes as per your instant pot.
4) After this time, carefully release the pressure of cooker, garnish with thyme and serve.

Recipe 02: Yummy Chicken Fajita

Freestyle Smart Points: 0
Total Time: 40 minutes
Servings: 4

Ingredients:

- 1 sliced onion
- 1 pound skinless and boneless lean chicken breasts, chop into strips
- 1 sliced bell pepper
- 1 cubed ripe tomato
- 2 teaspoons dry garlic powder
- 1 tablespoon ground cumin
- 1 teaspoon dry onion powder
- 1 teaspoon ground black pepper
- 1 teaspoon pink salt
- 1/2 teaspoon or more chili powder

Directions:

1) Preheat your oven to 375°F.
2) Spray a casserole dish with olive oil.
3) Mix seasoning together in a bowl.
4) Chop chicken into 1-inch bite-sized strips or pieces and coat them well with some seasoning blend.
5) Spread seasoned chicken pieces in a layer in the base of greased casserole dish.
6) Top chicken with vegetables. Bake at precisely 375°F for 35 to 40 minutes to brown vegetables.
7) Serve with tomato, lettuce, sour cream, guacamole, cheese, salsa, and tortillas.

Recipe 03: Yummy Baked Salmon

Freestyle Smart Points: 0, 6 ounces serving
Total Time: 20 minutes
Servings: 4

Ingredients:

- 3 minced garlic cloves
- 2 pounds salmon
- 1/4 cup chopped parsley
- Salt, to taste
- 1/2 cup shredded parmesan cheese

Directions:

1) Preheat your oven to 425°F.
2) Line your baking sheet with a parchment paper.
3) Season salmon filet with salt to taste.
4) Put salmon filet (skin-side down) on the parchment paper. Cover it with another parchment paper. Put fish in the oven to bake for almost 10 minutes.
5) Blend the minced garlic, parmesan cheese and chopped parsley in a bowl.
6) Take out salmon from oven and discard the top parchment paper.
7) Top salmon with herb mixture and put in the oven again. Cook for extra five minutes until done.
8) Take out from oven and wait for five minutes, serve hot.

Recipe 04: Delicious Chicken Nuggets

Freestyle Smart Points: 3 for each serving
Total Time: 30 minutes
Servings: 4

Ingredients:

- 1/2 cup whole wheat or all-purpose flour
- 1 pound skinless and boneless chicken breasts
- 20 mini pretzels or pretzel sticks
- 1/4 cup milk, skim
- 1/2 teaspoon black pepper
- 1 teaspoon garlic powder
- 1/4 cup brown spicy mustard

Directions:

1) Preheat your oven to 400°F.
2) Add pretzels in a zippered plastic bag and seal. Crush them with the help of one rolling pin, food processor or heavy glass.
3) Use three shallow containers for the creation of dredging station.
4) Put flour with garlic and pepper in a container. Put mustard and milk in another container. Put crushed pretzels in the final container.
5) Chop chicken into small bite-sized pieces.
6) Dredge pieces of chicken in flour, mustard and finally in the pieces of pretzel.
7) Put on one baking sheet and bake for almost 20 to 23 minutes to make nuggets. Serve hot.

Recipe 05: Chicken Verde in Crockpot

Freestyle Smart Points: 0, per serving
Total Time: 6 hours
Servings: 6

Ingredients:

- 2 seeded jalapenos
- 1 pound chicken breasts without skin and bone
- 1/2 white quartered onion
- 6 quartered and peeled tomatillos
- 2 minced garlic cloves
- 1/2 cup low sodium and fat-free chicken broth
- 1/2 teaspoon pink salt
- 1 teaspoon cumin seeds
- 1/4 teaspoon ground black pepper

Directions:

1) Puree jalapenos, quartered onion, tomatillos, garlic clove, pink salt, cumin seeds, ground black pepper and chicken broth in a blender to make it slightly chunky.
2) Put chicken in the base of the crockpot and add puree over chicken.
3) Cook this blend over low heat for almost 6 hours.
4) Shred chicken after six hours and serve with additional sauce over it.

Recipe 06: Zesty Chickpea Salad

Freestyle Smart Points: 0, 1/2 cup serving
Total Time: 10 minutes
Servings: 8

Ingredients:

- 30 ounces rinsed and drained chickpea
- 1 chopped tomato
- 1/2 teaspoon brown sugar
- 1/4 cup chopped onion
- 1/4 cup feta cheese, crumbled and reduced fat
- 1/2 tablespoon red vinegar
- 1/2 tablespoon fresh lemon juice
- 2 minced garlic cloves
- 1/4 teaspoon pepper
- 1/4 teaspoon salt
- 1 to 2 tablespoons cilantro
- 1 tablespoon Greek Yogurt

Directions:

1) Drain chickpeas and rinse thoroughly. Put them in a bowl.
2) Toss in tomato, brown sugar, onion, cheese, vinegar, lemon juice, garlic, pepper, salt, cilantro, and yogurt. Mix all ingredients well.
3) Now serve instantly and put the leftover in your fridge. You can secure it for a few days in your refrigerator.

Recipe 07: Grilled Shrimps with Tangy Sauce

Freestyle Smart Points: 0 per serving
Total Time: 20 minutes
Servings: 5

Ingredients:

- 2 tablespoons vinegar, balsamic
- 24 deveined and clean medium shrimp
- 1 lemon, for juice
- 1 teaspoon coconut or olive oil
- 1 clove minced garlic
- 1/2 teaspoon black pepper
- 1/2 teaspoon salt
- 1 pinch flakes of red pepper
- Sauce:
- 1 tablespoon Greek Yogurt
- 2 tablespoons tomato ketchup
- 1 tablespoon horseradish prepared sauce

Directions:

1) Take a bowl and mix together pepper flakes, pepper, salt, garlic, lemon juice, oil, and vinegar together.
2) Pour this blend over shrimp and cover shrimps to put in the fridge for almost 30 minutes.
3) Slide all shrimps (one by one) on skewers.
4) Carefully grill every side for 2 to 3 minutes. Shrimps take less time to cook so keep an eye on them when they turn pink and curl.
5) Sauce:
6) Take a bowl and mix ketchup, Greek yogurt, and horseradish sauce. You can increase or decrease horseradish sauce as per your taste.

Recipe 08: Steamed Asparagus Salad

Freestyle Smart Points: 0
Total Time: 10 minutes
Servings: 4

Ingredients:

- Asparagus stalks (peeled and trimmed): 1 pound
- Olive oil (extra-virgin): 2 tablespoons
- Ground pepper and Kosher salt as per taste
- Lemon Wedges: 1 lemon

Directions:

1) Pour almost 1" water in one large saucepan and set one inflatable steamer inside. Let this water boil and add the asparagus pieces in your steamer.
2) Cover this steamer and steam asparagus to make it crispy. It will take almost 4 - 5 minutes. Transfer all asparagus pieces into the heated dish for serving and drizzle with olive oil.
3) Sprinkle pepper and salt as per taste and garnish with fresh lemon wedges. Serve immediately.
4) You can sprinkle grated lemon zest and unsalted butter along with minced parsley leaf and oil.

Recipe 09: Stir-fried Chicken Salad

Freestyle Smart Points: 2
Total Time: 35 minutes
Servings: 4 servings

Ingredients:

- Chicken breasts (without bones and skin): 1 pound
- Minced garlic: 2 cloves
- Peeled ginger (matchsticks slices): 1 piece (2-inch)
- Soy sauce: 1 tablespoon
- Sugar: 1 tablespoon
- Cornstarch: 1 tablespoon + 1 teaspoon
- Kosher salt: 1-1/4 teaspoons
- Dry sherry: 1 tablespoon
- Chicken broth (zero sodium): 3/4 cup
- Vegetable oil: 2 tablespoons
- Asparagus (2 pounds): 2 bunches (trim woody stems and make 1-inch pieces)
- Scallions (green and white parts, thin slices): 1 bunch

Directions:

1) Keep chicken breasts for almost 20-30 minutes and make thin slices of chicken. Take a bowl and mix in chicken, ginger and garlic, sugar, soy sauce, salt (1 teaspoon), sherry and sugar (1 teaspoon). Marinate all these ingredients at your room temperature for almost 15 minutes. Stir in remaining cornstarch and broth in a separate bowl. Keep this bowl aside.

2) Take a nonstick skillet and heat one tablespoon oil over high flame. Add scallions, garlic, asparagus, salt (1/4 teaspoons), water (1/4 cup) and ginger in this pan. Stir fry these ingredients for almost three minutes and transfer in one bowl.

3) Heat one tablespoon oil in the same skillet and add chicken to stir-fry it for almost three minutes. Add the asparagus (in bowl) to this pan and mix to heat these ingredients well. Mix in the reserved mixture of corn starch and let it boil and reduce heat to simmer. You have to make it thick. Mound stir-fry ingredients on your serving plate and serve with brown rice.

Recipe 10: Egg and Potato Salad

Freestyle Smart Points: 2
Cooking Time: 10 minutes
Servings: 4

Ingredients:

- Boiled Potatoes (chopped): 4
- Olive oil: 2 tablespoons
- Lemon juice: 1/2 lemon
- Chopped parsley: 1 handful
- Boiled eggs: 2
- Wild rocket: 1 cup
- Diced cucumber: 1

Directions:

1) Take one bowl and toss boiled potatoes with parsley, lemon juice and olive oil in this bowl.
2) Stir in chopped boiled eggs and mix rocket leaves and diced cucumber to serve.

Recipe 11: Asparagus and Chicken Salad

Freestyle Smart Points: 2
Cooking Time: 30 minutes
Servings: 4

Ingredients:

- Vegetable oil: 3 tablespoons
- Hard-boiled eggs: 4
- Black pepper (ground): as per taste
- Chopped garlic: 2 cloves
- Asparagus (3-inch pieces): 1 pound
- Lemon (sliced): 1
- Slat: 1/2 teaspoon

Directions:

1) Heat some oil in a skillet over medium heat and cook garlic in hot oil for one minute. Season with salt, add asparagus, cover this skillet with one lid, and cook for 5 minutes. Stir frequently to avoid burning. Turn off heat.
2) Slowly mix quarter eggs in cooled asparagus blend, season with salt and pepper and garnish with slices of lemon.

Recipe 12: Zesty Asparagus Soup

Freestyle Smart Points: 4
Total Time: 30 minutes
Servings: 4

Ingredients:

- Butter: 25g
- Vegetable Oil: a little
- Asparagus spear (discard woody ends and chop stalks and tips, keep tips separate): 350g
- Shallow (Fine slices): 3
- Crushed garlic: 2 cloves
- Spinach: 2 handfuls
- Vegetable stock: 700ml
- Olive oil to drizzle
- Rustic bread: to serve

Directions:

1) Take one large saucepan and heat oil and butter in this pan. Fry tips of asparagus for a few minutes to make them soft. Transfer them to a plate and keep it aside.
2) Add asparagus stalks, garlic and shallots in similar pan and cook for almost 10 minutes. Mix in spinach and stock. Let them boil and blitz with one hand blender.
3) Sprinkle pepper and salt and pour hot water as per your need. Ladle this blend into bowls and sprinkle asparagus tips in each bowl. Drizzle with oil and serve with rustic bread.

Chapter 7 – WW Freestyle Dessert Recipes

Weight Watchers Freestyle plan allows you to enjoy delicious desserts during your diet. See these healthy and tasty recipes.

Recipe 01: Applesauce Cookies

Freestyle Smart Points: 4 per cookie
Total Time: 17 minutes
Servings: 24

Ingredients:

- 1/2 cup applesauce, unsweetened
- 1 sugar-free cake mix, yellow
- 2 eggs
- 1 cup diced apple
- 1/2 teaspoon ground cinnamon

Directions:

1) Preheat your oven to almost 375°F.
2) Line your baking sheet with parchment paper or silicone mats.
3) Take a bowl and combine cinnamon, apple, eggs, applesauce and cake mix in this bowl. Mix well to combine.
4) Scoop 1-inch balls on your baking sheet with 2" distance.
5) Bake in your preheated oven for 10 to 12 minutes, or until done.

Recipe 02: Cinnamon Muffins

Freestyle Smart Points: 3 per muffin
Total Time: 23 minutes
Servings: 18

Ingredients:

- 1-1/2 cups chopped apples
- 1 yellow or white cake mix, sugar-free
- 1 ripe banana, small
- 1/2 cup applesauce, unsweetened
- 2 teaspoons cinnamon powder
- 1 cup fresh water

Directions:

1) Preheat your oven to precisely 375°F.
2) Spray full-sized muffin cups or tins with a nonstick spray.
3) Take a bowl and mash banana in the bowl. Stir in water and applesauce and mix well.
4) Take a large bowl and mix in cinnamon and cake mix in this bowl.
5) Pour applesauce and banana blend into the cake mix blend. Mix well.
6) Fold in apples. Pour almost 1/4 cup batter into every muffin tin. You have to make 18 tins.
7) Bake in your preheated oven for almost 18 minutes or golden brown.
8) The middle of muffins should be moist, but free from liquid.

Recipe 03: Delicious Mint Fluff

Freestyle Smart Points: 3 per serving
Total Time: 35 minutes
Servings: 6

Ingredients:

- 2 cup cool whip, fat-free
- 8 ounces softened cream cheese, fat-free
- 1/4 teaspoon peppermint extract
- Chocolate chips
- Green food color, gel
- One pinch vanilla

Directions:

1) Mix cool whip, cream cheese, vanilla extract and peppermint extract in a bowl.
2) Add gel coloring (one drop at a time to reach the desired color) and mix well. Keep it in the fridge for 30 minutes before serving.
3) Top with some chocolate chips and serve with Graham crackers.

Recipe 04: Tasty Jello Cookies

Freestyle Smart Points: 2 per cookies
Total Time: 22 minutes
Servings: 24

Ingredients:

- 1 cup Splenda
- 2-1/2 cups all-purpose flour
- 1/2 cup Greek Yogurt, nonfat
- 2 eggs
- 1/4 cup melted butter
- 0.30 ounces sugar-free gelatin
- 2 teaspoons baking powder
- 1 teaspoon pure vanilla extract
- 1 teaspoon pink salt
- 1 tablespoon colorful sprinkles

Directions:

1) Preheat your oven to almost 350°F and line 2 to 3 cookie sheets with parchment paper or silicone mats for baking.
2) Take a bowl and whisk Splenda, vanilla extract, yogurt, eggs, and butter together in this bowl until smooth.
3) Slowly sift gelatin powder, salt, baking powder and flour in a bowl.
4) Stir well to form a dough and fold in sprinkles.
5) Use spoonfuls to drop batter on greased cookie sheets.
6) Bake for almost 10 to12 minutes in your preheated oven. Serve hot or cold.

Recipe 05: Healthy Ice cream

Freestyle Smart Points: 1 for each serving
Total Time: 30 minutes
Servings: 2

Ingredients:

- 3 sliced bananas
- 1 teaspoon pure vanilla extract
- 1/4 cup coconut or almond milk
- 4 tablespoons powdered cocoa

Directions:

1) Blend all ingredients in your food processor to make a smooth blend and combine everything.
2) Pour this blend into one dish and let it freeze for one hour. Serve chilled.

Recipe 06: Tangy Applesauce

Freestyle Smart Points: 0 per serving
Total Time: 30 minutes
Servings: 4

Ingredients:

- 1/4 cup brown sugar
- 4 apples, chopped, peeled and cored
- 1/5 teaspoon cinnamon powder
- 3/4 cup fresh water

Directions:

1) Combine cinnamon, sugar, water, and apples in a pan. Cover this pan and cook ingredients over medium flame for almost 15 – 20 minutes until tender.
2) Let it cool and use a potato masher or fork to mash this blend. Applesauce is ready.

Recipe 07: Baked Pears with Honey and Walnut

Freestyle Smart Points: 2, each pear
Total Time: 30 minutes
Servings: 2

Ingredients:

- 2 teaspoons honey
- 1/4 teaspoon ground cinnamon
- 2 ripe pears
- 1/4 cup walnuts, crushed
- Yogurt, optional

Directions:

1) Preheat your oven to precisely 350°F.
2) Cut pears in half and put pears on one baking sheet. You can cut the silver part off.
3) Use one melon baller or measuring spoon to scoop out seeds.
4) Now sprinkle some cinnamon and top with some walnuts. Drizzle almost 1/2 teaspoon of honey over each pear.
5) Bake in your oven for 30 minutes. Take it out, let the pears cool and serve.

Recipe 08: Butter Cookie

Freestyle Smart Points: 2
Total Time: 15 minutes
Servings: 4

Ingredients:

- 2 tablespoons soft butter
- 2 teaspoons olive oil
- 1/2 cup sugar (dark brown)
- 1 teaspoon strawberry (extract)
- 1/8 tsp salt
- Egg white (1 Egg)
- 3/4 cups flour (Flour)
- 1/4 teaspoon baking soda
- 3 oz chocolate chips (semi-sweet)

Directions:

1) Prepare your oven at 375 degrees F (190 degrees C). Prepare the blend of butter, oil, cream, and brown sugar.
2) Transfer salt, egg white, and strawberry extract and mix them properly. Mix the flour and baking soda in the mixture of cream and fold all the ingredients well.
3) You can add chocolate chips and mix for even distribution. Distribute the batter on the baking sheet evenly to make small balls. Always use a greased baking sheet. It will take 4 to 6 minutes to bake the cookies.

Recipe 09: Caramelized Apples

Freestyle Smart Points: 5
Total Time: 30 minutes
Servings: 2

Ingredients:

- 1/3 cup brown sugar
- 1/4 cup water
- 2 teaspoons low-fat butter
- 2 medium apples
- 2 tablespoons low-fat yogurt (vanilla flavored)
- 2 teaspoons chopped walnut

Directions:

1) Take brown sugar, water, and low-fat butter in a small cooking pot and bring these ingredients to a boiling point. Make it slightly thicker and then remove the cooking pot from heat.
2) Now keep this pot aside and cut the apples in half after peeling it. Arrange half parts of apple and reduce their size.
3) Drizzle the mixture of caramel on the apples and keep the tray in the oven to bake at 350 degrees.
4) Bake it for 25 minutes with cover, and then uncover it to bake for almost 25 minutes. Top the apples with yogurt after keeping in the dessert dishes. Add caramel and almonds as well.

Recipe 10: Potato and Apple Tart

Freestyle Smart Points: 5 (1/4 of tart in one serving)
Total Time: 1 hour 30 minutes
Servings: 4

Ingredients:

- 4 chopped potatoes
- 1 chopped apple
- 1 chopped onion
- 2 tablespoons chopped parsley
- 1/2 teaspoon salt
- 2 tablespoons olive oil
- 1/2 cup grated cheese – gruyere

Directions:

1) Heat an oven at almost 425 degrees Fahrenheit and grease a baking pan with edible olive oil. Now add potatoes, apple, onion, olive oil, parsley, pepper and salt in a large brown and mix them well.
2) Now pour half of this mixture in the baking pan and sprinkle a 1/4 th cup of cheese. Now pour remaining half of the cheese layer and cover the cake with a greased aluminum foil to maintain moisture.
3) Bake for 40 minutes and then remove foil and sprinkle 1/4 cup of remaining cheese. Bake it for another 15 minutes and cut into equal slices to enjoy

Recipe 11: Asparagus Smoothie

Freestyle Smart Points: 0
Total Time: 10 minutes
Servings: 1

Ingredients:

- Carrot juice: 1/2 cup
- Mango Pulp: 1 mango
- Chopped asparagus (broiled or cooked): 1 cup
- Avocado: 1/2 cup
- Ice cubes

Direction:

1) Take one smoothie blender and put all ingredients in this blender.
2) Carefully blend all ingredients and pour into the glass after getting desired consistency.

Recipe 12: Nutty Smoothie

Freestyle Smart Points: 5
Total Time: 10 minutes
Servings: 1

Ingredients:

- Coconut Milk: 1 cup
- Nuts (almonds and walnuts): 1/2 cup
- Chopped asparagus (broiled or cooked): 1 cup
- Dates (pitted): 1/2 cup
- Ice cubes

Directions:

1) Take one smoothie blender and put all ingredients in this blender.
2) Carefully blend all ingredients and pour into the glass after getting desired consistency.

Chapter 8 – Bonus WW Freestyle Recipes

Some bonus WW freestyle recipes can enhance the taste of your food. Here are some delicious dips and crespelle.

Recipe 01: Light Crespelle

Freestyle Smart Points: 1 for each
Total Time: 35 minutes
Servings: 20

Ingredients:

- 1-1/2 cups milk, 1%
- 1 cup whole wheat white flour
- 1 large egg
- 2 egg whites
- 1 teaspoon oil
- Olive oil to spray
- 1/2 teaspoon salt

Directions:

1) Put milk, salt, oil, egg whites, egg and flour in a blender. Blend well.
2) Heat a non-stick 8-inch skillet over medium heat. Grease pan with olive oil and pour almost two tablespoons of crespelles mixture in the pan. Slowly swirl this mixture around your pan to cover equally. Cook for nearly 30 seconds.
3) Flip to other side and cook for 10 seconds.
4) Remove crespelle and transfer on one plate. Replicate this procedure with remaining batter.

Recipe 02: Marinara Sauce

Freestyle Smart Points: 0 for half cup
Total Time: 30 minutes
Servings: 6

Ingredients:

- 2 cloves smashed garlic
- 1 teaspoon olive oil
- 1 bay leaf
- 28 ounces crushed tomatoes
- 1 teaspoon oregano
- Fresh pepper and salt, to taste
- 2 tablespoons chopped basil

Directions:

1) Heat 1-teaspoon olive oil in a pot over medium flame.
2) Add garlic in hot oil and sauté until golden, be careful to avoid burning.
3) Stir in oregano, bay leaf, pepper, salt, and crushed tomatoes. Mix well and decrease heat to almost low.
4) Cover this pot with a lid and let it simmer for almost 15 to 20 minutes.
5) Turn off heat and mix in fresh basil.

Recipe 03: Horseradish Sauce

Freestyle Smart Points: 0
Total Time: 5 minutes
Servings: 8

Ingredients:

- 3 tablespoons mayonnaise, reduced-fat
- 2 tablespoons homemade Prepared horseradish
- 1/8 teaspoon red pepper, ground
- 1 tablespoon apple cider vinegar
- 1/2 cup sour cream, nonfat
- 1 teaspoon powdered mustard

Directions:

1) Take a bowl and whisk together sour cream, ground pepper, mayonnaise, mustard, vinegar, and horseradish in this bowl. The sauce is ready.

Recipe 04: Pizza Sauce

Freestyle Smart Points: 0, per serving
Total Time: 40 minutes
Servings: 4

Ingredients:

- 6 ounces tomato paste
- 6 fluid ounces 110°F warm water
- 1/4 teaspoon oregano, dried
- 1/4 teaspoon marjoram, dried
- 1/4 tablespoon basil, dried
- 3 tablespoons parmesan cheese, grated
- 1/4 teaspoon black pepper, ground
- 1 teaspoon garlic, minced
- 1/8 teaspoon powdered cayenne pepper
- 2 tablespoons organic honey
- 1/8 teaspoon red pepper dried flakes
- teaspoon anchovy paste
- 3/4 teaspoon dried onion powder
- Salt as per taste

Directions:

1) Combine salt, red pepper flakes, cayenne pepper, black pepper, basil, marjoram, oregano, onion powder, anchovy paste, honey, garlic, parmesan cheese, water, and tomato paste in a bowl. Mix well and break up bunches of cheese.
2) The sauce must sit for almost 30 minutes to blend all flavors and spread it over pizza dough to prepare pizza as per your desire.

Recipe 05: Cranberry Sauce

Freestyle Smart Points: 0 per serving
Total Time: 10 minutes
Servings: 11

Ingredients:

- 12 oz. cranberries
- 1 cup brown sugar
- 1 cup fresh orange juice

Directions:

1) Take a pan and dissolve sugar in orange juice in this pan. Mix in cranberries and cook for almost 10 minutes until cranberries begin to pop.
2) Turn off heat and put the sauce in one bowl. Let it cool and serve.

Recipe 06: Prepared Horseradish

Freestyle Smart Points: 0 per serving
Total Time: 20 minutes
Servings: 1-1/2 cups

Ingredients:

- 8 tablespoons white vinegar
- 1 pound horseradish
- 2-1/2 teaspoons pink salt

Directions:

1) Peel horseradish root and coarsely grate it. Combine white vinegar (2 tablespoons), grated horseradish and pink salt in a food processor. Pulse 4 – 5 times to break horseradish down.
2) Stir in 6 tablespoons vinegar (one by one) and mix to form a coarse paste. Transfer this blend to one jar and put in the fridge for almost 1 month.

Recipe 07: Tangy BBQ Sauce

Freestyle Smart Points: 0, per serving
Total Time: 10 minutes
Servings: 12

Ingredients:

- 3 tablespoons brown sugar
- 1/2 cup tomato ketchup
- 1 teaspoon pink salt
- 1 teaspoon red chili powder
- 1/2 cup fresh water
- 1/4 cup apple cider vinegar

Directions:

1) Take a bottle or bowl and combine chili powder, salt, sugar, water, ketchup and vinegar in this bottle.
2) Shake well to mix and put in the fridge until you are ready to use.

Recipe 08: Pomegranate Dressing

Freestyle Smart Points: 2
Cooking Time: 15 minutes
Servings: 4

Ingredients:

- Pomegranate Juice: 4 tablespoons
- Olive oil: 4 tablespoons
- White vinegar: 2 tablespoons
- Caster sugar: 1/2 teaspoon
- Pomegranate seeds: 1/2 pomegranate

Directions:

1) Take one bowl, whisk all ingredients in this bowl, put this mixture in one jam jar, and shake it well.
2) The dressing is ready; you can keep it in your fridge for five days.

Recipe 09: Seasoning Mix

Freestyle Smart Points: 0
Cooking Time: 10 minutes
Servings: 15

Ingredients:

- Cornstarch: 1 tablespoon
- Salt: 1 teaspoon
- Paprika: 1 teaspoon
- Chili powder: 2 teaspoons
- Sugar: 1 teaspoon
- Onion powder: 1/2 teaspoon
- Chicken bouillon (crushed) cubes: 3/4 teaspoon
- Garlic powder: 1/4 teaspoon
- Cumin: 1/4 teaspoon
- Cayenne pepper: 1/4 teaspoon

Directions:

1) Mix all the ingredients in a bowl and select an airtight container to store it in a cool place.
2) You can use this seasoning in your fajita recipes.

Recipe 10: Pumpkin Pie Spice

Freestyle Smart Points: 0
Cooking Time: 10 minutes
Servings: 15

Ingredients:

- Ground allspice: 1 tablespoon
- Ground cinnamon: 1/4 cup
- Ground ginger: 4 teaspoons
- Ground nutmeg: 4 teaspoons

Directions:

1) Combine nutmeg, cinnamon, allspice and ginger together in a bowl.
2) You can use an airtight container to store it.

Conclusion

Weight Watchers Freestyle is a new and transformed addition to current WW programs. It allows you to enjoy plenty of free food items. You can enjoy these items in unlimited quantities. Typical programs of Weight Watchers work on a point system. Each food has particular points that are known as SmartPoints. While following Weight Watchers freestyle diet, you will be allocated specific points on a regular basis. You have to follow these points to portion your regular food.

This book is designed for your assistance with some weight watchers freestyle recipes. These recipes are available with points so that you can easily follow your designated points. You can follow the sample meal plan of this book or substitute some meals as per your choice. Stay Healthy!

CPSIA information can be obtained
at www.ICGtesting.com
Printed in the USA
LVHW100731210221
679518LV00014B/835